The 2024 Healthy Weight Loss Guide for women

A Woman's Essential Guide to Losing Weight and Keeping It Off in 2024

Betty B. Burton

Table of Contents

Introduction

Dear Reader,

Have you ever looked in the mirror and felt a wave of frustration wash over you? The image reflecting at you, a reminder of the unfulfilled promises you made to yourself year after year, seems to ask, "When will you finally feel confident and comfortable in your skin?"

If you're anything like the countless women I've had the privilege to work with, you know that the quest for a healthier, happier, and more vibrant you is not just about numbers on a scale or the latest diet trend. It's about reclaiming the life you deserve, rediscovering your self-worth, and embracing the journey towards a better you. It's about feeling that undeniable sense of confidence when you walk into a room, and knowing that you are radiating health and vitality.

"The 2024 Healthy Weight Loss Guide for Women" is not just another diet book. It's a roadmap, a companion, and a sanctuary for women from all walks of life who have yearned for real, lasting change. It's about rewriting your story, where the protagonist isn't a number on a scale, but a powerful, resilient woman who is ready to rewrite her narrative.

In the pages that follow, you'll find a guide that goes beyond the usual platitudes and one-size-fits-all solutions. This book is a love letter to every woman who has ever felt defeated by weight loss struggles, societal pressures, or the seemingly unattainable standards of beauty. It's an invitation to take a deep breath, shake off the past, and embrace the transformative potential within you.

We'll explore the latest research, practical strategies, and a mindset shift that will empower you to make 2024 the year you not only lose weight but keep it off for good. We'll address the mental and emotional aspects of the journey, acknowledging that a healthy lifestyle is as much about nurturing your spirit as it is about nourishing your body. This isn't just a book; it's a promise of support and guidance as you embark on this remarkable journey of self-discovery and transformation. It's a testament to the belief that every woman is capable of reaching her goals and living the life she desires.

So, are you ready to let go of self-doubt and embrace the path to a healthier, happier, and more confident you in 2024? Turn the page and let's begin this journey together.

Chapter 1

Setting the Foundation

Assessing Your Health Goals

In the journey to a healthier, happier you, the first step is the most pivotal one. Imagine embarking on a cross-country road trip without a destination in mind. You wouldn't know which roads to take, what sights to see, or when to celebrate your progress. In a way, your health goals are the destination on your path to well-being. But they're not just any destination; they're your treasure, the key to unlocking your best self. In this chapter, we'll help you map out your journey by diving deep into the vital process of assessing your health goals. Let's begin this transformative adventure with clarity, purpose, and enthusiasm.

The foundation of any successful endeavor is built on a solid understanding of your goals. When it comes to achieving a healthier lifestyle, setting clear, realistic, and sustainable health goals is essential. In this chapter, we'll guide you through the process of assessing your health goals, ensuring that they align with your unique desires and needs.

Why Assessing Your Health Goals Matters

Before you set out on your journey, it's crucial to answer the question, "Why?" Why do you want to achieve a healthier weight and a more vibrant life? Your "why" is your driving force, your source of motivation, and your anchor when the waters get rough.

Your reasons may be deeply personal – wanting to feel more confident, be more active with your family, or simply to lead a longer more fulfilling life. Or perhaps it's a vision of the future you, a self-assured and empowered woman radiating health and vitality. Your "why" is the heartbeat of your journey, so it's worth taking the time to listen to it.

Defining S.M.A.R.T. Goals

To ensure your health goals are effective and attainable, it's essential to make them S.M.A.R.T. – Specific, Measurable, Achievable, Relevant, and Time-bound.

1. Specific: Clearly define what you want to achieve. Rather than a vague goal like "I want to lose weight," specify, "I want to lose 15 pounds."

2. Measurable: You need a way to track your progress. If your goal is quantifiable, like the number of pounds or inches, you'll know when you've achieved it.

3. Achievable: While big dreams are wonderful, it's important to make sure your goals are within your reach. Set challenging but realistic targets.

4. Relevant: Your goals should be meaningful and aligned with your values and aspirations. They need to matter to you.

5. Time-bound: Set a deadline for when you intend to achieve your goal. This adds a sense of urgency and helps you stay on track.

The Power of Visualization

Close your eyes and picture yourself living your healthier, happier life. See yourself making better food choices, enjoying invigorating workouts, and exuding confidence. Visualization can be a potent tool for motivation and keeping your "why" in focus.

Action Steps for Assessing Your Health Goals

1. Take a moment to reflect on your "why." Write it down and revisit it whenever your motivation wanes.

2. Define your S.M.A.R.T. goals. Be specific about what you want to achieve, how you'll measure it, and when you'll accomplish it.

3. Create a vision board or journal where you can visualize your success. It can serve as a daily reminder of your aspirations.

4. Stay open to adjustments. As you progress, your goals might evolve. Flexibility is a key to long-term success.

Remember, the path to a healthier you is a journey, not a destination. Embrace the process, trust in your ability to change, and always stay connected to your "why." Your goals are not just about shedding pounds; they're about gaining a life filled with energy, confidence, and vitality. So let's take the first steps together, fueled by your dreams and guided by your unique goals. The road ahead is full of possibilities, and you are well on your way to realizing them.

Understanding Your Body's Needs

Understanding your body's needs is like deciphering the owner's manual to your unique, incredible machine. To embark on a successful journey to a healthier you, it's essential to speak your body's language, recognize its cues, and provide it with what it craves for optimal functioning. In this chapter, we'll delve into the intricacies of understanding your body's needs, from nourishment to hydration, and explore how to build a harmonious relationship with your body.

Nourishing Your Body: The Basics

Your body is an intricate network of systems, each with its own set of requirements. Proper nutrition is the fuel that keeps these systems running smoothly. When you nourish your body with the right foods, you're not just feeding it; you're investing in your long-term health and vitality.

1. Macronutrients: These are the building blocks of your diet: carbohydrates, proteins, and fats. Understanding the balance between them is key. Carbs provide energy, proteins support muscle growth and repair, and healthy fats are essential for various bodily functions.

2. Micronutrients: These include vitamins and minerals, which are equally vital. They regulate various bodily processes, such as immune function, metabolism, and bone health. A balanced diet ensures you get all the micronutrients your body needs.

3. Fiber: Fiber aids digestion, keeps you feeling full and helps manage blood sugar levels. It's abundant in fruits, vegetables, whole grains, and legumes.

4. Hydration: Water is the elixir of life. Staying adequately hydrated supports every bodily function, from digestion to temperature regulation. Aim for at least eight glasses of water a day.

Listening to Your Body

Your body is an amazing communicator. It tells you when it's hungry, when it's full, and when it needs specific nutrients. Tuning in to these signals is crucial for maintaining a healthy weight.

1. Hunger cues: Learn to distinguish between true hunger and emotional eating. When you're genuinely hungry, your body will send signals like stomach growling and feelings of emptiness. Respond to these cues with nourishing, balanced meals.

2. Fullness cues: Recognize the signs that your body has had enough to eat, such as a feeling of satisfaction, a pause in eating, or a decrease in the desire for more food.

3. Cravings: Understand that cravings are not necessarily your body's need for nutrients. They can be influenced by emotions, habits, or external cues. When a craving strikes, pause and ask yourself if it's true hunger or a desire for comfort or distraction.

Tailoring Your Diet to Your Body's Needs

Your body's needs are unique to you. Factors like age, gender, activity level, and any underlying health conditions will influence your nutritional requirements. Here's how to customize your diet:

1. Caloric needs: Calculate your daily caloric needs based on your goals, whether it's weight loss, maintenance, or muscle gain. It's important to strike a balance between energy intake and expenditure.

2. Meal planning: Structure your meals to provide a steady source of energy throughout the day. This may include smaller, more frequent meals or three well-balanced main meals.

3. Special dietary considerations: If you have specific dietary restrictions or health conditions, consult with a healthcare professional or registered dietitian to ensure you're meeting your body's needs.

Action Steps for Understanding Your Body's Needs

1. Keep a food diary for a week to track your eating habits. This will help you identify patterns and areas for improvement.

2. Educate yourself about macronutrients, micronutrients, and their food sources.

3. Pay close attention to your hunger and fullness cues during meals.

4. Stay hydrated throughout the day, making water your beverage of choice.

5. Consider consulting with a registered dietitian to create a personalized nutrition plan that aligns with your body's unique needs.

Understanding your body's needs is a cornerstone of your journey to a healthier lifestyle. By nourishing your body with the right foods, listening to its signals, and customizing your diet, you'll be well on your way to achieving your health goals. In the next chapter, we'll explore practical strategies for crafting a balanced meal plan that caters to your individual needs and preferences.

Building a Mindset for Success

In the journey to a healthier you, your mindset is your compass, your guiding star. It's the force that propels you forward when motivation wanes and obstacles arise. While we often focus on physical aspects, the power of your mind is the true driving force behind long-term success. In this chapter, we'll delve into building a mindset for success, exploring how your thoughts, beliefs, and attitudes can shape your journey to a healthier, happier you.

The Power of a Positive Mindset

Your mindset is a collection of your thoughts and beliefs. A positive mindset can be your greatest ally, while a negative one can be your harshest critic. Consider these factors:

1. Belief in Yourself: Believe that you have the ability to change and achieve your health goals. Self-doubt is a roadblock on your path to success.

2. Optimism: Cultivate an optimistic outlook. Optimism can enhance your resilience and make it easier to bounce back from setbacks.

3. Self-Compassion: Be kind to yourself. Mistakes and slip-ups are part of any journey. Treat yourself with the same kindness and encouragement you'd offer a close friend.

Embracing the Growth Mindset

A growth mindset is the belief that abilities and intelligence can be developed through effort, learning, and persistence. Embracing a growth mindset can revolutionize your approach to change.

1. Viewing Challenges as Opportunities: Instead of shying away from challenges, view them as opportunities for growth. Overcoming obstacles is where the most significant transformation happens.

2. Embracing Continuous Learning: Understand that you can always learn and improve. Whether it's trying a new exercise, exploring healthier recipes, or understanding the science of nutrition, a curious mind is a powerful asset.

Overcoming Limiting Beliefs

Our minds often hold us back with limiting beliefs. These may include "I've tried and failed before," "I'm not strong enough," or "I don't have time." Identifying and challenging these beliefs is a crucial step in building a success-oriented mindset.

Setting Realistic Expectations

It's important to set realistic expectations for your journey. Rapid, dramatic changes can be unsustainable and demotivating. Aiming for gradual, consistent progress is more likely to lead to long-term success.

Visualizing Success

Visualization is a powerful tool for building a success-oriented mindset. Envision yourself achieving your health goals in vivid detail. This not only provides motivation but also helps your brain align with your desired outcome.

Action Steps for Building a Mindset for Success

1. Keep a journal to track your thoughts and feelings regarding your health journey. Identify any negative or limiting beliefs.

2. Challenge these beliefs by seeking evidence to the contrary. For instance, if you believe you're not strong

enough, recall instances where you displayed resilience and strength.

3. Surround yourself with positive influences, whether it's supportive friends and family, inspirational books, or online communities.

4. Practice self-compassion. When you face challenges or setbacks, speak to yourself with kindness and encouragement.

5. Visualize your success regularly. Create a mental image of the healthier, happier you and return to it whenever motivation wanes.

A mindset for success is the cornerstone of your journey to a healthier lifestyle. By cultivating positive beliefs, embracing a growth mindset, and challenging limiting beliefs, you'll be better equipped to overcome obstacles and stay motivated.

It's the force that propels you forward when motivation wanes and obstacles arise.

Chapter 2

Nutrition Essentials

Navigating 2024's Dietary Trends

In a world where dietary trends come and go like the seasons, it can be challenging to decipher the best approach to nutrition. The abundance of information can lead to confusion and frustration. But fret not, for in this chapter, we will navigate the ever-changing landscape of dietary trends in 2024 and equip you with the knowledge to make informed, sustainable choices when it comes to nourishing your body.

The Dietary Landscape

The dietary landscape has evolved over the years, and 2024 brings with it a variety of approaches to nutrition, each claiming to be the key to health and weight management. From plant-based diets to intermittent fasting, ketogenic eating to paleo principles, it's a smorgasbord of options.

Finding Your Dietary Style

The truth is, there's no one-size-fits-all approach to nutrition. What works for one person may not work for another. It's essential to find a dietary style that aligns with your individual preferences, lifestyle, and health goals.

Balanced Nutrition: The Foundation

No matter which dietary trend you may choose to follow, a few fundamental principles remain consistent:

1. Variety: A diverse diet ensures you get a wide range of nutrients. Aim to incorporate different fruits, vegetables, whole grains, lean proteins, and healthy fats into your meals.

2. Portion Control: Even the healthiest foods can contribute to weight gain if consumed in excessive quantities. Be mindful of portion sizes to maintain a healthy balance.

3. Moderation: Enjoying your favorite treats is a part of a healthy diet. It's all about moderation. Occasional indulgences can be a part of a balanced eating plan.

Plant-Based Eating

The plant-based diet trend has gained considerable attention, with a focus on whole, plant-derived foods. This style of eating can offer various health benefits, from weight management to reduced risk of chronic diseases. Whether you choose to go completely plant-based or adopt a flexitarian approach, plants should play a significant role in your diet.

Intermittent Fasting

Intermittent fasting is another trend on the rise. It involves cycling between periods of eating and fasting. The key is not only when you eat but also what you eat during your eating window. It can be an effective strategy for weight management and metabolic health.

Ketogenic and Low-Carb Diets

Low-carb diets, including the ketogenic diet, emphasize reducing carbohydrate intake to promote fat-burning for energy. These diets can be effective for some people, particularly those with specific health conditions. However, they may not be suitable for everyone.

Paleo and Whole Foods Approach

The paleo diet and a focus on whole foods have gained popularity as well. The idea is to consume foods that our ancestors would have eaten, which typically excludes processed foods. It can be a valuable approach for those seeking to eliminate processed and unhealthy options.

Action Steps for Navigating Dietary Trends

1. Consider your personal preferences, dietary restrictions, and health goals when evaluating dietary trends.

2. Experiment with different approaches, but give each one time to see how your body responds. What works for you is what matters most.

3. Consult with a registered dietitian or healthcare professional for personalized guidance based on your specific needs.

4. Remember that balance, variety, portion control, and moderation are key principles of a healthy diet, regardless of the trend you choose.

In 2024, navigating dietary trends is about finding a nutritional style that suits you and your unique goals. The journey to a healthier you involves understanding the ever-evolving dietary landscape, making informed choices, and adapting your approach as needed. In the following chapters, we'll delve deeper into crafting a balanced meal plan that aligns with your chosen dietary style and helps you reach your health objectives.

Crafting a Balanced Meal Plan

As you embark on your journey to a healthier lifestyle, crafting a balanced meal plan is like drawing the blueprint for your daily nourishment. A well-balanced diet is not only essential for weight management but also for overall health, energy, and vitality. In this chapter, we'll guide you through the art of creating a meal plan that is both nutritious and satisfying, allowing you to achieve your health goals with ease.

The Building Blocks of a Balanced Meal

A balanced meal is a symphony of nutrients that provides your body with the energy and nourishment it needs. It typically consists of three essential components:

1. Protein: Protein is the foundation of every meal. It supports muscle growth and repair, helps you feel full, and stabilizes blood sugar levels. Include lean sources like poultry, fish, tofu, legumes, or lean cuts of meat.

2. Carbohydrates: Carbohydrates provide the energy your body craves. Opt for complex carbohydrates such as whole grains, vegetables, and fruits, which offer fiber and sustained energy.

3. Fats: Healthy fats are essential for various bodily functions, including brain health and hormone production. Include sources like avocados, nuts, seeds, and olive oil in your meals.

The Plate Method

A simple yet effective way to create balanced meals is by using the plate method. Here's how it works:

- Fill half of your plate with non-starchy vegetables like leafy greens, broccoli, or bell peppers. These provide essential vitamins and fiber.
- Reserve a quarter of your plate for lean protein, such as chicken, fish, or plant-based options like tofu or legumes.
- Use the remaining quarter for complex carbohydrates like brown rice, quinoa, or whole-grain pasta.
- Add a small serving of healthy fats, like a drizzle of olive oil or a sprinkle of nuts.

Snacking Smartly

Snacks can be part of a balanced meal plan, too. Opt for nutrient-dense snacks like Greek yogurt, fresh fruit, or a handful of almonds. These keep your energy levels stable between meals and prevent excessive hunger.

Meal Timing and Frequency

In addition to what you eat, when and how often you eat also matters. Aim to:

- Have regular, balanced meals to maintain stable blood sugar levels and curb overeating.
- Include a source of protein in every meal, as it helps keep you full.
- Eat mindfully, savoring each bite and paying attention to your body's hunger and fullness cues.

Customizing Your Meal Plan

Your balanced meal plan should align with your dietary style and individual preferences. Whether you follow a plant-based diet, embrace intermittent fasting, or have specific dietary restrictions, you can customize your meals to suit your needs.

Action Steps for Crafting a Balanced Meal Plan

1. Start by planning your meals for the week, taking into account your dietary style and personal preferences.

2. Experiment with new recipes and ingredients to keep your meals exciting and enjoyable.

3. Use the plate method as a visual guide to ensure balanced meals.

4. Pay attention to portion sizes to avoid overeating.

5. Stay flexible and open to adjustments in your meal plan as you learn more about what works best for your body.

Crafting a balanced meal plan is not just about eating to lose weight; it's about nourishing your body for a healthier, more vibrant life. With the right balance of protein, carbohydrates, and healthy fats, you'll be better equipped to reach your health goals and maintain your well-being. In the upcoming chapters, we'll explore effective exercise routines, stress management, and other elements that, when combined with a balanced meal plan, will contribute to your path to a healthier you.

Superfoods and Their Impact

In the ever-evolving world of nutrition, the term "superfoods" has gained immense popularity. These are foods that are touted for their exceptional nutrient content and potential health benefits. While there's no magical solution to health, understanding the impact of superfoods and incorporating them into your diet can offer significant advantages on your journey to a healthier you. In this chapter, we'll explore the concept of superfoods and how they can positively influence your health and well-being.

Defining Superfoods

Superfoods are nutrient-dense foods packed with vitamins, minerals, antioxidants, and other beneficial compounds. They are often associated with health-promoting properties, from supporting heart health to reducing the risk of chronic diseases.

The Impact of Superfoods

1. Antioxidant Power: Many superfoods are rich in antioxidants, which help combat oxidative stress and reduce inflammation in the body. Antioxidants can contribute to overall well-being and have been linked to a lower risk of chronic diseases.

2. Heart Health: Several superfoods, such as berries, fatty fish, and nuts, are known for their heart-protective properties. They can help lower cholesterol levels, reduce blood pressure, and support overall cardiovascular health.

3. Brain Function: Superfoods like leafy greens, fatty fish, and berries are associated with improved cognitive function and a reduced risk of age-related cognitive decline.

4. Weight Management: Some superfoods are low in calories but high in fiber and nutrients, making them excellent choices for those looking to manage their weight. They help you feel full and satisfied without excess calories.

5. Gut Health: Foods like yogurt, kefir, and fermented vegetables contain probiotics, which support a healthy gut microbiome. A balanced gut microbiome is essential for digestion, immunity, and overall health.

Common Superfoods and Their Impact

1. Berries: Blueberries, strawberries, and raspberries are packed with antioxidants and have been linked to improved brain function and reduced oxidative stress.

2. Fatty Fish: Salmon, mackerel, and sardines are rich in omega-3 fatty acids, which support heart health and may reduce the risk of chronic diseases.

3. Leafy Greens: Spinach, kale, and Swiss chard are abundant in vitamins and minerals, supporting overall health and well-being.

4. Nuts and Seeds: Almonds, walnuts, chia seeds, and flaxseeds provide healthy fats, fiber, and a range of nutrients, contributing to heart health and weight management.

5. Yogurt: Probiotic-rich yogurt supports gut health and digestion, and it is a good source of calcium and protein.

6. Legumes: Beans, lentils, and chickpeas are high in fiber and protein, making them valuable for weight management and overall health.

Incorporating Superfoods into Your Diet

Incorporating superfoods into your diet is a practical way to enhance your nutrition and overall health. Here are some tips:

1. Add berries to your morning cereal or yogurt for a burst of antioxidants.

2. Include fatty fish like salmon in your weekly meals.

3. Experiment with leafy greens in salads, smoothies, or as a side dish.

4. Snack on a handful of nuts and seeds for a satisfying, nutrient-rich treat.

5. Enjoy yogurt with fresh fruit or as a base for smoothies.

6. Incorporate legumes into soups, stews, or salads for added fiber and protein.

Action Steps for Superfoods and Their Impact

1. Identify superfoods that align with your dietary preferences and health goals.

2. Gradually introduce these superfoods into your meals and snacks, experimenting with recipes and flavors.

3. Be mindful of portion sizes, as even superfoods can contribute to excess calorie intake when consumed in large quantities.

4. Consult with a registered dietitian for personalized guidance on incorporating superfoods into your diet effectively.

Superfoods are like nutritional powerhouses that can positively impact your health and well-being. While they won't magically transform your health overnight, integrating them into your diet as part of a balanced meal plan can support your journey to a healthier you. In the following chapters, we'll continue to explore essential elements of a healthy lifestyle, including exercise, stress management, and more, to provide you with a holistic approach to well-being.

Chapter 3

Exercise and Movement

Tailoring Workouts for Women

Exercise is not a one-size-fits-all endeavor, and it certainly isn't limited to a specific gender. However, understanding that women have unique physiological, hormonal, and practical considerations when it comes to exercise is crucial for tailoring effective workout routines. In this chapter, we'll explore the world of exercise and movement, focusing on how to customize workouts to meet the specific needs and goals of women.

The Benefits of Exercise for Women

Regular physical activity offers a myriad of benefits for women, including:

1. Weight Management: Exercise helps burn calories and build lean muscle, contributing to weight control and management.

2. Cardiovascular Health: Aerobic exercise can reduce the risk of heart disease, lower blood pressure, and improve cholesterol levels.

3. Mood and Stress Management: Physical activity releases endorphins, reducing stress and enhancing mood, making it a powerful tool for managing daily pressures.

4. Bone Health: Weight-bearing exercises, such as walking and strength training, support bone health and can help prevent osteoporosis.

5. Hormonal Balance: Exercise can regulate hormonal imbalances, alleviate symptoms of premenstrual syndrome (PMS), and contribute to a healthier menopausal transition.

Customizing Workouts for Women
When tailoring workouts for women, consider the following factors:

1. Hormonal Fluctuations: Understand how the menstrual cycle can affect energy levels and motivation. Adjust workout intensity and type based on where you are in your cycle.

2. Strength Training: Incorporate resistance training into your routine to build lean muscle, increase metabolism, and enhance bone health. Don't be afraid of weights; they are essential for women.

3. Cardiovascular Exercise: Include aerobic workouts like running, swimming, or dancing for heart health and calorie burning. Adjust the intensity based on your fitness level and goals.

4. Core and Pelvic Floor Health: Focus on exercises that strengthen the core and pelvic floor, especially during and after pregnancy. These muscles provide essential support for overall well-being.

5. Flexibility and Mobility: Incorporate stretching and mobility exercises to maintain flexibility and prevent injuries. Yoga and Pilates can be particularly beneficial.

Postpartum Exercise

For women who have recently given birth, postpartum exercise is a unique consideration. It's essential to start gradually, listening to your body and seeking guidance from a healthcare professional. Pelvic floor exercises, gentle core work, and low-impact activities can help you regain strength and fitness safely.

Practical Tips for Women's Workouts

1. Set Realistic Goals: Establish clear, achievable fitness goals that align with your lifestyle and time constraints.

2. Mix It Up: Variety keeps exercise enjoyable and prevents plateaus. Incorporate a mix of cardio, strength, and flexibility training into your routine.

3. Listen to Your Body: Pay attention to how your body responds to exercise. If you're fatigued or experiencing discomfort, adjust your workout accordingly.

4. Stay Consistent: Consistency is key. Even on busy days, find ways to incorporate movement, whether it's a quick walk or a few minutes of stretching.

5. Seek Professional Guidance: Consider consulting a fitness trainer, physical therapist, or certified postnatal specialist for personalized advice and guidance.

Exercise is a powerful tool for women's health, offering a wide range of physical and emotional benefits. Tailoring workouts to address the unique needs and goals of women can help you maximize the advantages of physical activity. In the upcoming chapters, we'll delve into the importance of the mind-body connection, stress management, and the practical aspects of sustaining a healthy lifestyle.

Embracing Effective Exercise Routines

Effective exercise routines are the heart and soul of a healthy lifestyle. Whether you're new to fitness or looking to revamp your current approach, understanding the key principles of creating effective workout plans is essential. In this chapter, we'll explore the world of exercise routines and how to embrace them in a way that maximizes your fitness gains and overall well-being.

The Pillars of Effective Exercise Routines

1. Consistency: Consistency is the cornerstone of any successful exercise routine. Regular, ongoing physical activity is essential for achieving and maintaining your fitness goals. Whether it's daily, several times a week, or with planned rest days, creating a consistent schedule is crucial.

2. Variety: Your body thrives on variety. Incorporating different types of exercises, such as cardiovascular, strength training, flexibility, and balance work, can prevent plateaus, reduce the risk of overuse injuries, and keep your workouts engaging.

3. Progression: As your fitness level improves, it's important to progress your workouts to continue challenging your body. This can be done by increasing weights, reps, or intensity. Progressive overload is the key to ongoing results.

4. Balance: Effective routines strike a balance between different forms of exercise. Cardiovascular workouts help burn calories and boost heart health, while strength training builds lean muscle, increases metabolism, and enhances bone health. Flexibility and balance exercises contribute to overall mobility and injury prevention.

5. Listening to Your Body: Pay close attention to your body's signals. If you're feeling fatigued, it's okay to take a rest day or opt for a lighter workout. Pushing through pain or exhaustion can lead to burnout or injuries.

Effective Cardiovascular Exercise

Cardiovascular exercise, often known as "cardio," is integral to any effective workout routine. It elevates your heart rate, burns calories, and strengthens your cardiovascular system. Options include running, cycling, swimming, dancing, and brisk walking. Customize your cardio routine based on your fitness level, interests, and goals.

Strength Training for Lean Muscle

Strength training is essential for building and maintaining lean muscle mass. It helps boost your metabolism, increase bone density, and enhance functional strength. Incorporate compound exercises like squats, deadlifts, and bench presses, as well as isolation exercises for specific muscle groups.

Flexibility and Balance Work

Don't overlook flexibility and balance exercises. These routines improve joint mobility, reduce the risk of injuries, and help you move with ease. Yoga and Pilates are excellent choices for enhancing flexibility and balance.

Embracing Effective Exercise Routines

1. Set Clear Goals: Define your fitness goals, whether they are weight loss, muscle gain, improved endurance, or overall well-being. Having a clear objective will guide your exercise routine.

2. Plan and Schedule: Create a weekly exercise schedule that incorporates cardiovascular, strength, and flexibility workouts. Make exercise a non-negotiable part of your day.

3. Seek Professional Guidance: Consider working with a fitness trainer or joining exercise classes to ensure proper form and technique. This can also provide accountability and motivation.

4. Track Your Progress: Keep a fitness journal to track your workouts, including the exercises, sets, reps, and weights. This will help you see your progress and identify areas for improvement.

5. Stay Motivated: Find activities you enjoy, work out with a buddy for added motivation, or reward yourself for achieving fitness milestones.

Action Steps for Embracing Effective Exercise Routines

1. Create a detailed exercise plan that includes the types of workouts, frequency, and duration.

2. Customize your workouts to suit your fitness level and goals.

3. Progress your workouts as you get stronger and fitter.

4. Make exercise a non-negotiable part of your routine, and find ways to stay motivated and accountable.

Effective exercise routines are the foundation of a healthier, happier you. By embracing workouts that are consistent, varied, progressive, and well-balanced, you can achieve and maintain your fitness goals while enjoying the physical and mental benefits of regular physical activity. In the following chapters, we'll delve into the mind-body connection, stress management, and the importance of maintaining long-term well-being.

Integrating Activity into Daily Life

Incorporating physical activity into your daily life isn't just about structured workouts; it's about embracing movement as a fundamental part of your daily routine. In this chapter, we'll explore the importance of integrating activity into your everyday life, offering practical strategies to keep you moving, healthy, and energized.

The Sedentary Lifestyle Conundrum

In our modern world, sedentary lifestyles have become all too common. Many of us spend prolonged hours sitting at desks, in front of screens, or during commutes. This sedentary behavior can lead to a host of health issues, from weight gain to musculoskeletal problems and an increased risk of chronic diseases.

Why Integrate Activity Daily?

1. **Counteracting Prolonged Sitting:** By integrating movement into your day, you can counteract the negative effects of sitting for extended periods.

2. **Weight Management:** Regular, low-intensity activities help burn extra calories and support weight management.

3. Energy and Focus: Movement can boost your energy levels and improve focus and productivity.

4. Stress Relief: Physical activity serves as a natural stress reliever, reducing tension and promoting a sense of well-being.

Practical Strategies for Integrating Activity

1. Take Active Breaks: Stand up, stretch, or take short walks during work breaks. Even a few minutes of movement can break up prolonged sitting.

2. Use the Stairs: Opt for stairs over elevators whenever possible. Climbing stairs is an excellent form of exercise.

3. Walking Meetings: Instead of sitting in a conference room, conduct walking meetings. It's a productive way to integrate movement and brainstorm creatively.

4. Park Farther Away: When going to work or running errands, park your car farther from your destination. The extra walking adds up.

5. Active Commuting: Consider walking or biking to work if the distance allows. Alternatively, use public transportation and walk to and from transit stops.

6. Home Exercises: Perform quick, home-based exercises during your daily routine. For instance, do squats while waiting for your coffee to brew or perform lunges while brushing your teeth.

7. Standing Workstation: If feasible, invest in a standing workstation to reduce the time spent sitting during work hours.

8. Gardening: Gardening is a productive way to stay active while enjoying the outdoors. It's a great way to burn calories and improve mood.

9. Family Activities: Include your family in your quest for more activity. Go for family walks, bike rides, or play active games together.

The Power of Consistency

The key to integrating activity into your daily life is consistency. Small, regular bursts of activity can add up to significant health benefits over time. By moving a habit, you can reap the rewards of better health, increased vitality, and enhanced well-being.

Action Steps for Integrating Activity into Daily Life

1. Assess your daily routine to identify opportunities for additional activity.

2. Set achievable daily activity goals, such as taking a certain number of steps or incorporating specific movements into your routine.

3. Track your progress to stay accountable and motivated.

4. Share your goals with a friend or family member to keep each other motivated.

5. Gradually build up the duration and intensity of your integrated activities as your fitness level improves.

Integrating activity into your daily life is a powerful way to maintain health, counteract the negative effects of prolonged sitting, and enjoy increased vitality. By making small, consistent changes to your daily routine, you can improve your physical and mental well-being, one step at a time.

Chapter 4

Mind-Body Connection

Stress Management and Weight Loss

The intricate relationship between your mind and body plays a significant role in your overall well-being. When it comes to weight management, stress can be a hidden saboteur. In this chapter, we'll delve into the mind-body connection, explore how stress affects weight, and provide practical strategies for managing stress to support your weight loss goals.

The Mind-Body Connection

The mind and body are deeply intertwined, and each can influence the other. Stress, in particular, can have a profound impact on your physical health. When you experience stress, your body releases hormones like cortisol and adrenaline, which can trigger a cascade of physiological responses. These responses can lead to emotional eating, cravings for comfort foods, and changes in metabolism, ultimately affecting your weight.

Stress and Emotional Eating

Stress often leads to emotional eating as a coping mechanism. When stressed, many people turn to food for comfort. High-calorie, sugary, or fatty foods can provide a temporary sense of relief and pleasure, but they can also contribute to weight gain over time.

Cortisol and Weight Gain

The stress hormone cortisol plays a significant role in weight management. Elevated cortisol levels are associated with increased fat storage, particularly in the abdominal area. This not only affects body weight but also raises the risk of chronic diseases.

Stress-Related Lifestyle Habits

Stress can also influence other lifestyle habits that impact weight, such as disrupted sleep patterns, decreased physical activity, and irregular eating habits. These changes can further complicate weight management efforts.

Stress Management Strategies

Effectively managing stress is essential for weight loss and overall well-being. Here are practical strategies to incorporate into your routine:

1. Exercise: Physical activity is a powerful stress reliever. Regular workouts release endorphins, reduce cortisol levels, and improve mood.

2. Mindfulness and Meditation: These practices help you stay present, reduce anxiety, and manage stress. Even a few minutes of deep breathing or meditation can be highly beneficial.

3. Healthy Eating: Opt for nutritious foods that nourish your body and support stress management. Avoid excessive caffeine and alcohol, which can exacerbate stress.

4. Time Management: Organize your daily tasks and priorities to reduce stress. Avoid overloading your schedule and allocate time for relaxation and self-care.

5. Social Connections: Spend time with friends and loved ones. Social support is a powerful stress buffer.

6. Sleep Hygiene: Prioritize good sleep habits. Aim for seven to eight hours of quality sleep each night.

7. Professional Help: If stress becomes overwhelming and impacts your daily life, consider consulting a mental health professional for guidance and support.

Mind-Body Techniques for Stress Management

Mind-body techniques, such as yoga and tai chi, are exceptional ways to connect your mental and physical well-being. These practices combine physical postures, controlled breathing, and mindfulness to reduce stress, improve relaxation, and enhance overall health.

Action Steps for Stress Management and Weight Loss

1. Identify your primary stressors and triggers.

2. Create a daily routine that incorporates stress management strategies, such as exercise, meditation, and healthy eating.

3. Practice mindfulness and relaxation techniques to reduce the impact of stress on your eating habits.

4. Prioritize self-care and allocate time for activities that bring you joy and relaxation.

5. Seek professional help if stress becomes unmanageable or leads to unhealthy eating patterns.

Managing stress is an essential component of a successful weight loss journey. By understanding the mind-body connection, acknowledging the role of stress in weight gain, and implementing stress management strategies, you can support your physical and emotional well-being. In the upcoming chapters, we'll continue to explore essential elements of a holistic approach to well-being, providing you with the tools to achieve and maintain a healthier lifestyle.

Mindfulness and Its Role in Healthy Habits

Mindfulness is a powerful tool that can profoundly impact your relationship with food, eating habits, and overall well-being. In this chapter, we'll explore the concept of mindfulness and its significant role in cultivating healthy habits, promoting mindful eating, and supporting your journey to a healthier lifestyle.

Understanding Mindfulness

At its core, mindfulness is about being fully present in the moment, without judgment or distraction. It involves paying deliberate attention to your thoughts, emotions, and sensations as they arise. This practice can extend to all aspects of life, including eating.

The Role of Mindfulness in Healthy Habits

1. Mindful Eating: Mindful eating involves savoring each bite, chewing slowly, and paying attention to the flavors and textures of your food. This practice helps prevent overeating and promotes a healthier relationship with food.

2. Stress Reduction: Mindfulness can reduce stress and emotional eating by allowing you to acknowledge and manage your emotions without turning to food for comfort.

3. Improved Awareness: By cultivating awareness, you can recognize hunger and fullness cues, making it easier to eat by your body's needs.

4. Enhanced Enjoyment: Mindful eating allows you to truly enjoy your meals, savoring the experience of nourishing your body.

Practical Strategies for Mindful Eating

1. Eat Without Distractions: Avoid eating in front of the TV or computer. Instead, focus solely on your meal.

2. Chew Slowly: Take your time with each bite, savoring the flavors and textures. This not only enhances mindfulness but also aids digestion.

3. Listen to Your Body: Pay attention to your hunger and fullness cues. Eat when you're hungry, and stop when you're satisfied.

4. Be Present: Enjoy your meal without multitasking. Put away your phone and fully engage with the experience of eating.

5. Mindful Grocery Shopping: Plan your meals, make a shopping list, and stick to it. Avoid impulse purchases that may not align with your health goals.

Mindfulness in Daily Life

While mindfulness can have a significant impact on eating habits, its benefits extend beyond the dining table. By integrating mindfulness into your daily life, you can experience improved focus, reduced stress, and enhanced overall well-being.

Action Steps for Mindfulness and Healthy Habits

1. Start with small, manageable changes in your eating habits. Focus on one meal or snack at a time.

2. Practice mindful eating by paying attention to your food, chewing slowly, and savoring each bite.

3. Use mindfulness techniques to reduce stress and emotional eating, such as deep breathing or meditation.

4. Integrate mindfulness into your daily routine. Set aside time for mindfulness exercises, even if it's just a few minutes a day.

5. Cultivate self-compassion by being kind and patient with yourself as you develop these practices.

Mindfulness is a powerful tool that can reshape your relationship with food, reduce stress, and enhance your overall well-being. By practicing mindful eating and integrating mindfulness into your daily life, you can support your journey to a healthier lifestyle and cultivate lasting, healthy habits. In the following chapters, we'll explore additional elements of holistic well-being and provide you with a comprehensive approach to maintaining your health and vitality

The Power of Sleep for Weight Management

Sleep is a crucial yet often overlooked aspect of weight management and overall health. In this chapter, we'll explore the profound impact of sleep on your weight, metabolism, and overall well-being, emphasizing the importance of getting quality rest for a healthier lifestyle.

The Connection Between Sleep and Weight

Sleep plays a significant role in regulating various hormones and processes that impact your weight:

1. Hormonal Balance: Sleep is essential for maintaining hormonal balance, especially those that regulate hunger and appetite. Inadequate sleep can disrupt these hormones, leading to increased appetite and cravings for high-calorie foods.

2. Metabolism: Quality sleep is essential for a healthy metabolism. A lack of sleep can slow down your metabolic rate, making it more challenging to maintain or lose weight.

3. Blood Sugar Control: Poor sleep can impair your body's ability to regulate blood sugar, increasing the risk of insulin resistance and weight gain.

4. Emotional Regulation: Sleep is crucial for emotional well-being. Inadequate sleep can lead to increased stress, anxiety, and depression, which may trigger emotional eating and weight gain.

How to Prioritize Quality Sleep

1. Consistent Sleep Schedule: Go to bed and wake up at the same times each day, even on weekends. This helps regulate your body's internal clock.

2. Create a Relaxing Bedtime Routine: Engage in calming activities before bedtime, such as reading, meditation, or gentle stretching.

3. Optimize Your Sleep Environment: Make your bedroom conducive to quality sleep by keeping it dark, quiet, and at a comfortable temperature.

4. Limit Screen Time: Avoid screens, such as phones and computers, at least an hour before bedtime. The blue light emitted from screens can interfere with your sleep cycle.

5. Watch Your Diet: Avoid heavy meals and caffeine close to bedtime, as they can disrupt sleep. Alcohol can also impact sleep quality.

6. Regular Physical Activity: Regular exercise can promote better sleep. However, avoid vigorous workouts close to bedtime.

7. Stress Management: Practice stress-reduction techniques, such as mindfulness and deep breathing, to calm your mind before sleep.

The Sleep-Weight Connection in Action

1. Adequate Sleep Promotes Weight Loss: Getting enough quality sleep can support weight loss efforts by helping regulate hunger hormones and boosting metabolism.

2. Improved Emotional Well-Being: Quality sleep is essential for emotional well-being, reducing stress and emotional eating.

3. Stress Reduction: A good night's sleep enhances stress management, helping you stay focused and better equipped to cope with life's challenges.

Action Steps for Prioritizing Quality Sleep

1. Create a regular sleep schedule and stick to it.

2. Establish a calming bedtime routine to prepare your body for rest.

3. Optimize your sleep environment for comfort and tranquility.

4. Limit screen time before bedtime and avoid heavy meals and caffeine.

5. Engage in regular physical activity to support sleep quality.

6. Practice stress management techniques to ensure a calm and peaceful mind before sleep.

Quality sleep is a powerful tool for weight management and overall well-being. By understanding the connection between sleep and weight, prioritizing your sleep quality, and incorporating healthy sleep habits into your daily routine, you can significantly enhance your efforts toward a healthier lifestyle. In the upcoming chapters, we'll continue to explore other essential elements of holistic well-being, providing you with a comprehensive approach to maintaining your health and vitality.

Chapter 5

Lifestyle Changes and Long-Term Maintenance

Sustainable Habits for Lasting Results

Lasting results in weight management and overall health are achieved through sustainable lifestyle changes. In this chapter, we'll explore the importance of embracing sustainable habits, creating a supportive environment, and staying motivated to maintain your progress for the long term.

The Power of Sustainable Habits

Sustainable habits are the backbone of a healthy lifestyle. Unlike short-term diets or fads, these habits can be maintained for a lifetime, ensuring lasting results. Sustainable habits are not only good for weight management but also your overall health and well-being.

Embracing Sustainable Changes

1. Gradual Progress: Make changes at a pace that suits your lifestyle and preferences. Gradual changes are more likely to stick.

2. Balanced Nutrition: Focus on balanced, nutritious meals and portion control. Avoid extreme diets that are difficult to sustain.

3. Regular Physical Activity: Find activities you enjoy and can commit to regularly. Make exercise a part of your routine.

4. Mindful Eating: Continue practicing mindful eating to prevent overeating and enjoy your meals.

5. Quality Sleep: Prioritize sleep as an essential part of your daily routine for better health and weight management.

6. Stress Management: Continue to practice stress-reduction techniques to support emotional well-being and prevent emotional eating.

Creating a Supportive Environment

1. Surround Yourself with Positivity: Build a network of supportive friends and family who encourage your healthy habits.

2. Remove Temptations: Keep unhealthy foods out of your home to reduce the likelihood of indulging in them.

3. Plan Ahead: Prepare healthy meals and snacks in advance to avoid making poor choices when you're hungry and short on time.

4. Seek Professional Support: If necessary, consult with a registered dietitian, personal trainer, or mental health professional for guidance and support.

Staying Motivated for the Long Term

1. Set New Goals: Continually set new, achievable goals to keep your motivation high.

2. Track Your Progress: Maintain a journal or use apps to track your progress, celebrate your achievements, and identify areas for improvement.

3. Reward Yourself: Use non-food rewards to celebrate milestones and maintain motivation.

4. Stay Mindful: Continue to practice mindfulness in all aspects of your life to reduce stress and maintain emotional well-being.

5. Embrace Variety: Keep your routine fresh and engaging by trying new exercises and recipes to prevent boredom.

6. Celebrate Non-Scale Victories: Recognize the importance of non-scale achievements, such as increased energy, better mood, and improved overall health.

Action Steps for Sustainable Habits and Long-Term Maintenance

1. Reflect on the sustainable habits you've embraced so far and consider how they can be maintained for the long term.

2. Identify any areas where you may need to make adjustments to ensure the sustainability of your lifestyle changes.

3. Create a supportive environment that reinforces your healthy habits and eliminates potential obstacles.

4. Set new, motivating goals that excite you and keep you focused on your journey.

5. Continue practicing mindfulness and stress management to ensure emotional well-being.

Sustainable habits are the key to long-term success in weight management and overall health. By creating a supportive environment, staying motivated, and continuously adapting your routine, you can maintain your progress and enjoy a lifetime of well-being. In the upcoming chapters, we'll explore additional elements of holistic well-being, providing you with a comprehensive approach to maintaining your health and vitality.

Overcoming Plateaus and Challenges

On the path to a healthier lifestyle, plateaus and challenges are inevitable. In this chapter, we'll explore common obstacles, including weight loss plateaus, emotional challenges, and setbacks, and provide strategies to overcome them and stay on track toward your health and well-being goals.

Understanding Plateaus and Challenges

Plateaus and challenges are a natural part of any health and fitness journey. They can manifest in various forms, including weight loss plateaus, emotional hurdles, and periods of stagnation. Understanding that these obstacles are common and can be overcome is essential for long-term success.

Overcoming Weight Loss Plateaus

1. Reassess Your Habits: Reevaluate your nutrition and exercise routines. Are you still adhering to your sustainable habits, or have there been subtle deviations?

2. Change Up Your Workouts: Introduce new exercises or increase the intensity of your current ones. Your body may adapt to your routine, resulting in a weight loss plateau.

3. Revisit Your Caloric Intake: If you've been following a calorie-restricted diet, your metabolism may have adjusted to the lower intake. Consider a brief caloric increase or a refeed period to "reset" your metabolism.

4. Stay Patient and Persistent: Understand that plateaus are normal. Keep in mind that weight loss may not always be linear; there will be periods of stagnation, followed by progress.

5. Focus on Non-Scale Victories: Don't solely rely on the scale to measure your progress. Celebrate non-scale victories like improved energy, better sleep, and increased strength.

Addressing Emotional Challenges

1. Stress Management: When faced with emotional challenges, utilize stress management techniques such as mindfulness, deep breathing, or meditation to maintain emotional well-being.

2. Seek Support: Reach out to a friend, family member, or mental health professional to discuss your emotional challenges and gain perspective.

3. Mindful Eating: Continue practicing mindful eating to avoid emotional eating and address emotional triggers for unhealthy eating habits.

4. Self-Compassion: Be kind to yourself. Understand that setbacks and challenges are part of the journey. Approach yourself with self-compassion and avoid self-criticism.

Overcoming Setbacks

Setbacks are an inherent part of any journey toward improved health and well-being. Here's how to handle them:

1. Acknowledge and Learn: Recognize your setbacks without judgment. Reflect on what led to them and what you can learn from the experience.

2. Set New Goals: After a setback, set new, achievable goals to get back on track. This can reignite your motivation and enthusiasm.

3. Stay Persistent: Stay committed to your long-term goals. Don't let setbacks deter you from your overall mission.

4. Seek Support: If a setback feels particularly challenging, reach out for support from friends, family, or professionals who can help guide you through it.

Action Steps for Overcoming Plateaus and Challenges

1. Reflect on any plateaus, emotional challenges, or setbacks you've encountered on your journey.

2. Identify the specific challenges and obstacles you face.

3. Implement strategies to overcome these challenges based on the guidance provided.

4. Stay persistent, practice self-compassion, and seek support when needed.

Plateaus and challenges are a normal part of your journey to improved health and well-being. By understanding how to overcome them and using them as opportunities for growth and learning, you can continue to make progress and work toward your long-term goals.

Tools for Maintaining Weight Loss

Sustaining weight loss is a commendable achievement, but it requires ongoing effort and the right tools to maintain your success. In this chapter, we'll explore the essential tools and strategies for keeping the weight off and continuing to live a healthy and fulfilling life.

Lifelong Maintenance Tools

1. Mindfulness: Continue practicing mindfulness in your eating habits and daily life. This awareness of your body's signals, your emotions, and your environment can help prevent overeating and make healthier choices.

2. Regular Exercise: Maintain a consistent exercise routine that incorporates both cardiovascular workouts and strength training. Exercise not only helps you control your weight but also contributes to your overall well-being.

3. Nutrition Knowledge: Keep learning about nutrition, balanced eating, and portion control. Understanding the nutritional value of foods empowers you to make informed choices.

4. Stress Management: Stress can be a significant factor in weight management. Continue practicing stress reduction techniques, such as meditation, yoga, or deep breathing, to support emotional well-being.

5. Self-Care: Prioritize self-care as a non-negotiable part of your routine. Taking time for yourself, whether through relaxation, hobbies, or pampering, is essential for maintaining a healthy mindset.

6. Supportive Environment: Surround yourself with people who support your healthy lifestyle. Share your goals with friends and family, and seek their encouragement and understanding.

Continuous Goal Setting

Set new, meaningful goals to keep you motivated and on track. These goals could be related to fitness, nutrition, emotional well-being, or personal development. Having clear objectives helps maintain your focus and enthusiasm for a healthy lifestyle.

Mindful Eating Practices

Maintain your commitment to mindful eating. Eating slowly, savoring each bite, and listening to your body's hunger and fullness cues are habits that contribute to successful weight maintenance.

Regular Check-Ins

Regularly assess your progress and make any necessary adjustments to your lifestyle. Use tools such as journaling, apps, or consultations with health professionals to keep track of your habits and make informed decisions.

Support and Accountability

Consider joining a support group or working with a personal trainer, dietitian, or therapist as needed. Accountability can be a powerful motivator and guide navigating challenges.

Consistency and Adaptability

Maintain consistency in your healthy habits, but also be adaptable. Life is full of changes and challenges. It's essential to remain resilient and find creative solutions to stay on the path to well-being.

Non-Scale Victories

Continue to celebrate non-scale victories as a reminder of your progress. Improved energy, mood, confidence, and overall health are all significant achievements that should be acknowledged and appreciated.

Action Steps for Maintaining Weight Loss

1. Review the tools and strategies discussed in this chapter and identify those that are most relevant to your situation.

2. Set new, motivating goals for yourself that align with your long-term well-being.

3. Continuously practice mindfulness in your eating habits and daily life.

4. Conduct regular check-ins to assess your progress and make necessary adjustments.

5. Consider seeking support and accountability, whether through a group or professionals.

Maintaining weight loss is an ongoing journey that requires dedication and the right tools. By continuing to embrace a mindful, balanced, and active lifestyle, setting meaningful goals, and staying adaptable and resilient, you can enjoy the benefits of lasting weight management and a lifetime of well-being. In the concluding chapters, we'll provide additional insights and guidance for sustaining your health and vitality.

Chapter 6

External Support and Resources

Community and Support Systems

Building and maintaining a healthy lifestyle can be a challenging but highly rewarding journey. In this chapter, we'll explore the importance of external support and resources, including the power of community and support systems, in helping you stay motivated, overcome obstacles, and sustain your well-being goals.

The Value of Community and Support Systems

Humans are inherently social creatures, and having a sense of community and support is essential for overall well-being. When it comes to adopting and maintaining a healthier lifestyle, this support network becomes even more critical.

Types of Support Systems

1. Friends and Family: Your loved ones can provide invaluable support and encouragement on your journey.

They can be your cheerleaders, workout partners, and a source of motivation.

2. Support Groups: Joining a support group or community of individuals with similar goals can provide a sense of belonging and accountability. You can share experiences, challenges, and success stories with like-minded individuals.

3. Professional Guidance: Consult with registered dietitians, personal trainers, therapists, or other health professionals for expert advice, guidance, and personalized plans.

4. Online Communities: The internet offers a vast array of online forums, social media groups, and apps dedicated to health and fitness. These can provide a sense of community and resources for information and inspiration.

The Role of Community in Motivation

Being part of a supportive community can be a powerful motivator. Here's how community support can help:

1. Accountability: Knowing that others are aware of your goals and progress can hold you accountable for your actions.

2. Sharing Knowledge: Community members can share their experiences, tips, and resources to enhance your understanding of health and fitness.

3. Emotional Support: During times of challenge or setbacks, the empathy and encouragement from others can be comforting and uplifting.

Action Steps for Building a Support System

1. Identify Your Needs: Consider the types of support you need and the specific goals you want to achieve.

2. Engage with Supportive Communities: Seek out local or online groups that align with your interests and goals. Join these communities and start participating.

3. Share Your Journey: Be open and share your goals, challenges, and successes with your support system. This can foster a sense of accountability.

4. Be Supportive in Return: Offer support, encouragement, and motivation to others in your community. It's a two-way street, and your support can make a difference in someone else's journey.

The Power of Positive Influence

Being part of a supportive community can help you maintain a positive attitude and stay focused on your goals. Surrounding yourself with individuals who share your vision for a healthier lifestyle can be highly motivating.

Overcoming Obstacles Together

Challenges will arise on your journey to well-being. Your support system can provide valuable insights, strategies, and emotional support to help you overcome these obstacles. Remember, you are not alone in your pursuit of a healthier, happier life.

Sustaining Your Journey with Support

As you continue your journey toward a healthier lifestyle, remember that you don't have to do it alone. Embrace the power of community and support systems to stay motivated, learn from others, and overcome challenges together.

Technology and Apps for Weight Management

In today's digital age, technology and smartphone apps have become valuable tools for individuals seeking to manage their weight, improve their health, and sustain a healthier lifestyle. This chapter explores the role of technology and the numerous apps available for weight management and well-being.

The Digital Revolution in Weight Management

Technology has revolutionized the way we approach weight management. Smartphones, fitness trackers, and a multitude of apps have made it easier than ever to track your progress, access information, and stay motivated on your health journey.

Benefits of Using Technology and Apps

1. Tracking Progress: Apps can help you monitor your exercise routines, nutrition, and weight loss goals, providing a clear picture of your progress.

2. Education: Access to information on nutrition, exercise, and well-being is just a few taps away, empowering you with knowledge to make informed choices.

3. Motivation: Many apps offer features like goal setting, reminders, and rewards, helping you stay motivated and on track.

4. Accountability: Sharing your goals and progress with an online community or a friend can hold you accountable for your actions.

5. Personalization: Some apps use your data to provide personalized recommendations for nutrition and exercise, catering to your specific needs and preferences.

Types of Weight Management Apps

1. Calorie Tracking Apps: These apps help you log your food intake and track your calorie consumption. They can also provide nutritional information and meal planning.

2. Fitness Apps: Fitness apps offer exercise routines, guided workouts, and the ability to track your physical activity, such as step count, distance, and duration.

3. Mental Well-Being Apps: Stress management and mindfulness apps can aid in reducing emotional eating and improving emotional well-being.

4. Health and Wellness Trackers: These apps allow you to monitor various health metrics like weight, blood pressure, and sleep patterns.

5. Community Apps: Join online communities, support groups, or forums dedicated to health and fitness to share experiences, seek motivation, and find support.

Action Steps for Using Weight Management Apps

1. Identify Your Needs: Determine which aspects of your weight management journey could benefit from technology and apps. For example, if you struggle with calorie tracking, consider a calorie-counting app.

2. Research and Download: Explore app stores for options that match your needs. Read user reviews and consider trying a few different apps to see which works best for you.

3. Set Up Your App: Once you've chosen an app, set up your profile, input your goals, and begin tracking your progress.

4. Stay Consistent: Use the app consistently to record your data and monitor your progress. Consistency is key to achieving and maintaining results.

5. Explore Community and Support: If the app offers community features, consider joining or participating in these to enhance your motivation and accountability.

The Future of Weight Management Technology

As technology continues to advance, the capabilities of weight management apps are likely to expand. We can expect more personalized and data-driven solutions, enhanced user experiences, and the integration of artificial intelligence to offer tailored guidance.

Integrating Technology into Your Lifestyle

Incorporating technology and apps into your weight management journey can help you maintain a healthy lifestyle in the modern world. These tools offer convenience, motivation, and knowledge, ultimately empowering you to sustain your well-being goals. In the subsequent chapters, we'll delve into further aspects of holistic health and equip you with the tools you need to maintain your health and vitality.

Professional Guidance and Counseling

While the support of friends, family, and technology can be invaluable on your journey to weight management and well-being, there are times when seeking professional guidance and counseling becomes crucial. In this chapter, we'll explore the importance of working with experts in the field of health and well-being.

The Role of Professional Guidance

Professional guidance and counseling play a pivotal role in helping individuals navigate the complexities of weight management and overall health. These experts possess the knowledge, experience, and skills necessary to provide personalized guidance and support.

Types of Health Professionals

1. Registered Dietitians and Nutritionists: These experts can offer personalized nutrition plans, helping you make informed dietary choices, and ensuring you're receiving the necessary nutrients.

2. Personal Trainers: A personal trainer can develop an exercise plan tailored to your goals, fitness level, and any specific needs or limitations you may have.

3. Mental Health Professionals: Psychologists, therapists, and counselors specialize in addressing emotional and mental health issues, such as emotional eating, body image concerns, and stress management.

4. Health Coaches: Health coaches can provide holistic support, offering guidance on nutrition, exercise, stress management, and lifestyle changes.

When to Seek Professional Guidance

There are several situations where professional guidance is highly beneficial:

1. Complex Health Conditions: If you have complex health conditions, like diabetes, heart disease, or food allergies, professional guidance can help you manage your weight and health safely.

2. Significant Weight Loss Goals: If you have substantial weight loss goals, a registered dietitian or nutritionist can help you create a safe and effective plan.

3. Emotional Challenges: If emotional eating, stress, or mental health concerns are affecting your weight management efforts, a mental health professional can provide valuable support.

4. Fitness and Exercise: Personal trainers can assist in creating a workout plan that aligns with your goals and ensures that you exercise safely and effectively.

5. Plateaus and Challenges: When facing plateaus or obstacles in your weight management journey, experts can offer guidance to overcome these hurdles.

The Benefits of Professional Guidance

1. Personalized Plans: Professionals can create customized plans that take into account your unique needs, goals, and limitations.

2. Education: You'll gain a deeper understanding of nutrition, exercise, and stress management, enabling you to make informed choices.

3. Accountability: Regular sessions with a professional can help hold you accountable for your actions and progress.

4. Emotional Support: Mental health professionals can offer emotional support and strategies for managing stress and emotional eating.

Action Steps for Seeking Professional Guidance

1. Identify Your Needs: Determine which areas of your weight management journey could benefit from professional guidance.

2. Research and Select Professionals: Look for reputable experts in your area or consider online services.

3. Schedule an Appointment: Contact the professional you've chosen and schedule an initial appointment.

4. Share Your Goals and Concerns: In your sessions, be open and honest about your goals, challenges, and needs.

5. Implement Recommendations: Act on the guidance and recommendations provided by the professional to support your weight management and well-being goals.

The Value of Collaboration

Often, a multidisciplinary approach involving multiple professionals can yield the best results. For example, a team consisting of a registered dietitian, personal trainer, and mental health professional can address various aspects of your health and well-being comprehensively.

Professional Guidance as a Long-Term Resource

Professional guidance and counseling are not only beneficial in the short term but can serve as a valuable resource for long-term health and well-being. Regular sessions with these experts can help you navigate the evolving challenges and goals of your journey.

Building and maintaining a healthy lifestyle can be a challenging but highly rewarding journey.

Conclusion

In conclusion, "The 2024 Healthy Weight Loss Guide for Women: A Woman's Essential Guide to Losing Weight and Keeping It Off in 2024" is a comprehensive resource that empowers women to take control of their health and well-being. Throughout this book, we've explored a wide range of topics, from setting the foundation for a healthy lifestyle to embracing mindfulness, nutrition essentials, exercise, and the power of sleep.

We've discussed the significance of sustainable habits and the role of external support, including community, technology, and professional guidance. By delving into these areas, we've equipped readers with the knowledge and tools they need to embark on a journey of weight management and holistic well-being.

Weight management is not just about a number on the scale; it's about embracing a lifestyle that fosters lasting health, vitality, and self-confidence. It's about understanding your body's unique needs, nourishing it with the right foods, staying active, and cultivating a mindful approach to eating. It's about managing stress, seeking support, and using technology to your advantage. It's about recognizing that professional guidance can be a valuable resource and that building a supportive community can be your foundation for success.

As we close this chapter on your weight management journey, remember that the path to a healthier, happier you is ongoing. It's about persistence, resilience, and adaptability. It's about celebrating your victories, whether they're recorded on the scale or not, and continuously setting new, motivating goals to keep you moving forward.

By incorporating the knowledge and practices shared in this book into your daily life, you have the power to transform your relationship with your body and embrace a future full of health and vitality. Remember, it's not just about the year 2024; it's about the rest of your life. Your journey to a healthier you is an investment in a brighter, more fulfilling future.

Thank you for joining us on this journey, and may your path be filled with success, well-being, and an abundance of health for years to come.